INTRODUCTION

There are thousands of promises to be found in the Word of God. These promises were put there for you and me. They will meet every need we have while living on this earth. Therefore, it is very important for us to receive or possess these promises.

You may ask though, how do I possess these promises? The Bible tells us that "Death and life are in the power of the tongue" (Proverbs 18:21). What we say becomes a part of our lives, whether we are saying good or bad, or positive or negative things. So, we should be confessing over our lives those positive things that line up with the Word of God. The more we confess the promises of God, the quicker they will manifest themselves in our daily lives. The Bible also tells us to speak to the mountain (sickness, weakness, disease, poverty, confusion, pain, etc.) and tell the mountain where to go and stay (Mark 11:23). We continue to confess the promises found in the Word of God as we speak to the mountain until it leaves.

In most instances, the mountain will not leave instantly or overnight, but if you persist and keep speaking the Word (God's promises), the Word will manifest itself and the problem will leave.

Confess the promises that you need at least three times or more each day. Before very long, you will begin to believe in your heart what you are saying with your mouth, and then the promises will manifest themselves in your life. Allow yourself time to get going in this area. Remember, if you will stay consistent by speaking God's Word to the mountain, it will leave and your circumstances will conform to the Word of God.

By applying this principle of confessing God's promises each day, you will be able to maintain a life of victory. This will keep your faith level high, as well as prevent a lot of trouble from coming your way. When Satan attacks you in any area, you can instantly resist him with the promises of God. The sooner you resist the attack of the devil, the quicker it will leave.

Put your name or the name of the one you are praying for in each blank of every verse. Confess the promise out loud if you can. Confession can be made quietly to yourself when circumstances prevent you from speaking out loud. Remember, you can have what you say if you do not doubt in your heart, but believe that those things you say will happen (Mark 11:23)

4

DAILY RECORD OF MY CONFESSIONS

SINNER'S PRAYER
To Receive Jesus As Savior

Are you born again? Have you ever received Jesus as your Lord and Savior? If your answers to these questions are no, but you would like Jesus to be your Savior, read these Scriptures and pray this prayer, agreeing with it in your heart.

John 3:16 "For God so loved the world, that he gave his only begotten Son, that whosoever believeth in him should not perish, but have everlasting life."

Romans 10:9-10 & 13 "That if thou shalt confess with thy mouth the Lord Jesus, and shalt believe in thine heart that God hath raised him from the dead, thou shalt be saved. For with the heart man believeth unto righteousness; and with the mouth confession is made unto salvation. For whosoever shall call upon the name of the Lord shall be saved."

John 14:6 "Jesus said unto him, I am the way, the truth, and the life: no man cometh unto the Father, but by me."

PRAY THIS PRAYER Dear God in Heaven, I come to You believing that Jesus Christ died on the cross for man's sins. I open the door to my heart and invite Jesus to come in and be my personal Lord and Savior. Jesus, forgive me for all my sins and cleanse me from all unrighteousness. Teach me God's Word, and fill me with the power of Your Holy Spirit. Give me knowledge and wisdom, and show me how to live a victorious life. I thank You, Jesus, because I am born again and saved through Your shed blood on the cross at Calvary. I am on my way to heaven in the Name of Jesus.

RECEIVE THE FULLNESS OF THE HOLY SPIRIT

Acts 19:2 "Have ye received the Holy Ghost since ye believed?" It is important to receive this New Testament experience by making sure you are filled with the Holy Spirit. As believers, we should have the same experience with the Holy Ghost as they did in the Book of Acts. Acts 1:8 says, "But ye shall receive power..." We need the power of the Holy Ghost in our lives! Mark 16:17 says, "...In my name ... they shall speak with new tongues." In Luke 11:13 it says, "How much more shall your heavenly Father give the Holy Spirit to them that ask him?" Acts 2:38 tells us that after we are born again, we shall receive the gift of the Holy Ghost. In Acts 2:4, the 120 believers in the Upper Room were **all** filled with the Holy Ghost and began to speak with other tongues, as the Spirit gave them utterance.

Remember, God is no respecter of persons (Romans 2:11). This means that what He has done for anyone else, He will do for you. Now, ask your Heavenly Father, in the Name of Jesus, to baptize you or fill you with the fullness of the Holy Spirit. Go ahead and speak in your new prayer language! Now, keep yourself built up by praying in the Holy Ghost (Jude 20).

PRAYER Heavenly Father, I ask You to fill me with Your Holy Spirit. I receive Him by faith in the Name of Jesus. I thank You, Father, for filling me with the power and anointing of the Holy Spirit. Now, I will speak in other tongues, as the Spirit gives me the language in Jesus' Name.

HOW TO RECEIVE
GOD'S PROMISES

Put your name and the name of anyone else you are praying for in the blanks of each verse. Pray, confess and claim these promises three times or more each day until you have what you want from your heavenly Father. As you claim these promises in your daily walk with the Lord, they will help keep your faith strong and prevent the devil from putting sickness, disease or bondage on you.

GOD'S WORD

<u>**Promise 1**</u>   **Proverbs 4:20-23** My son (___), attend to my words; incline thine (___) ear unto my sayings. Let them not depart from thine (___) eyes; keep them in the midst of thine (___) heart. For they are life unto those (___) that find them, and health (and healing) to all their (___) flesh. Keep thy (___) heart with all diligence; for out of it are the issues of life.

I Peter 2:2 As newborn babes, desire the sincere milk of the word, that ye (___) may grow thereby.

Hebrews 4:12 For the word of God is quick, and powerful, and sharper than any twoedged sword, piercing even to the dividing asunder of (___) soul and spirit, and of the joints and marrow, and is a discerner of the thoughts and intents of (___) heart.

Job 22:28 Thou (___) shalt also decree a thing, and it shall be established unto thee (___): and the light shall shine upon thy (___) ways.

TONGUE-MOUTH
<u>Promise 2</u> **Proverbs 18:21** Death and life are in the power of the (___) tongue: and they (___) that love it shall eat the fruit thereof.

Proverbs 10:11 The mouth of a righteous man (___) is a well of life.

Mark 11:23-24 For verily I say unto you (___), That whosoever (___) shall say unto this mountain (problem), Be thou removed, and be thou cast into the sea; and shall not doubt in his (___) heart, but shall believe that those things which he (___) saith shall come to pass; he (___) shall have whatsoever he (___) saith. Therefore I say unto you (___), What things soever ye (___) desire, when ye (___) pray, believe that ye (___) receive them, and ye (___) shall have them.

Proverbs 12:18 But the tongue of the wise (___) is health (healing).

Peter 3:10 For he (___) that will love life, and see good days, let him (___) refrain his (___) tongue from evil, and his (___) lips that they speak no guile.

SALVATION - BORN AGAIN

Promise 3 **Romans 10:9-10 & 13** That if thou
(___) shalt confess with thy (___) mouth the Lord
Jesus, and shalt believe in thine (___) heart that
God hath raised him (Jesus) from the dead, thou
(___) shalt be saved. For with the heart man (___)
believeth unto righteousness; and with the mouth
(your mouth) confession is made unto salvation.
For whosoever (___) shall call upon the name of
the Lord (Jesus) shall be saved.

John 3:16 For God so loved the world (___), that
he gave his only begotten Son, that whosoever
(___) believeth in him should not perish, but have
everlasting life.

John 14:6 Jesus saith unto him (___), I am the
way, the truth, and the life: no man (___) cometh
unto the Father, but by me.

I John 5:12 He (___) that hath the Son hath life
and he (___) that hath not the Son of God hath no
life.

DELIGHT IN GOD'S WORD

<u>Promise 4</u> **Psalm 1:1-3** Blessed is the man (___) that walketh not in the counsel of the ungodly, nor standeth in the way of sinners, nor sitteth in the seat of the scornful. But his (___) delight is in the law of the Lord; and in his law doth he (___) meditate day and night. And he (___) shall be like a tree planted by the rivers of water, that bringeth forth his (___) fruit in his (___) season; his (___) leaf also shall not wither; and whatsoever he (___) doeth shall prosper.

II Timothy 2:15 Study to show thyself (___) approved unto God, a workman that needeth not to be ashamed, rightly dividing the word of truth (God).

Psalm 37:4 Delight thyself (___) also in the Lord; and he shall give thee (___) the desires of thine (___) heart.

Psalm 45:7 Thou (___) lovest righteousness, and hatest wickedness: therefore God, thy (___) God, hath anointed thee (___) with the oil of gladness above thy fellows.

I WILL NOT FEAR

Promise 5   **Psalm 27:1-5**   The Lord is my (___) light and my (___) salvation; whom shall I (___) fear? the Lord is the strength of my (___) life; of whom shall I (___) be afraid? When the wicked, even mine (___) enemies and my (___) foes, came upon me (___) to eat up my (___) flesh, they stumbled and fell. Though an host should encamp against me (___), my (___) heart shall not fear: though war should rise against me (___), in this will I be confident. One thing have I (___) desired of the Lord, that will I (___) seek after; that I (___) may dwell in the house of the Lord all the days of my (___) life, to behold the beauty of the Lord, and to inquire in his temple. For in the time of trouble he shall hide me (___) in his pavilion: in the secret of his tabernacle shall he hide me (___); he shall set me (___) up upon a rock.

Psalm 46:1   God is our (___) refuge and strength, a very present help in trouble.

II Timothy 1:7   For God hath not given us (___) the spirit of fear; but of power, and of love, and of a sound mind.

JESUS IS MY SHEPHERD

<u>Promise 6</u> **Psalm 23:1-6** The Lord is my (___) shepherd; I (___) shall not want. He maketh me (___) to lie down in green pastures: he leadeth me (___) beside the still waters. He restoreth my (___) soul: he leadeth me (___) in the paths of righteousness for his name's sake. Yea, though I (___) walk through the valley of the shadow of death, I (___) will fear no evil: for thou art with me (___); thy rod and thy staff they comfort me (___). Thou preparest a table before me (___) in the presence of mine (___) enemies: thou anointest my (___) head with oil; my (___) cup runneth over. Surely goodness and mercy shall follow me (___) all the days of my (___) life: and I (___) will dwell in the house of the Lord for ever.

Psalm 19:14 Let the words of my (___) mouth, and the meditation of my (___) heart, be acceptable in thy sight, O Lord, my (___) strength, and my (___) redeemer.

THANKSGIVING

<u>Promise 7</u>   **Philippians 4:6-7**   (___) be careful for nothing; but in every thing by prayer and supplication with thanksgiving let your (___) requests be made known unto God. And the peace of God, which passeth all understanding, shall keep your (___) hearts and minds through Christ Jesus.

Colossians 4:2   (___) continue in prayer, and watch in the same with thanksgiving.

Psalm 100:4   (___) enter into his gates with thanksgiving, and into his courts with praise: be thankful unto him, and bless his name.

Psalm 50:14   (___) offer unto God thanksgiving; and pay thy (___) vows unto the most High.

Psalm 69:30   I (___) will praise the name of God with a song, and will magnify him with thanksgiving.

Psalm 95:2   Let us (___) come before his presence with thanksgiving, and make a joyful noise unto him with psalms.

PRAISE

<u>Promise 8</u>   **Psalm 8:1-2** O Lord our (___) Lord, how excellent is thy name in all the earth! Who hast set thy glory above the heavens. Out of the mouth of (___) babes and sucklings hast thou ordained strength (praise Matt. 21:16) because of thine enemies, that thou mightest still the enemy (Satan, demons) and the avenger.

Psalm 34:1-4 I (___) will bless the Lord at all times: his praise shall continually be in my (___) mouth. My (___) soul shall make her boast in the Lord: the humble (___) shall hear thereof, and be glad. O magnify the Lord with me (___), and let us (___) exalt his name together. I (___) sought the Lord, and he heard me (___), and delivered me (___) from all my (___) fears.

Psalm 22:3   But thou art holy, O thou that inhabitest the praises of Israel (___).

Hebrews 13:15 By him (Jesus) therefore let us (___) offer the sacrifice of praise to God continually, that is, the fruit of our (___) lips giving thanks to his name.

PRAISE

<u>Promise 9</u> **Psalm 42:11** Why art thou cast down, O my (___) soul? And why art thou disquieted within me (___)? Hope thou in God: for I (___) shall yet praise him, who is the health of my (___) countenance, and my (___) God.

Psalm 100:1-5 (___) Make a joyful noise unto the Lord, all ye lands. Serve the Lord with gladness: come before his presence with singing. Know ye (___) that the Lord he is God: it is he that hath made us (___), and not we ourselves; we (___) are his people, and the sheep of his pasture. Enter into his gates with thanksgiving, and into his courts with praise: be thankful unto him, and bless his name. For the Lord is good; his mercy is everlasting; and his truth endureth to all (___) generations.

Psalm 9:1-2 I (___) will praise thee, O Lord, with all my (___) whole heart; I (___) will show forth all thy marvellous works. I (___) will be glad and rejoice in thee: I (___) will sing praise to thy name, O thou most High.

Psalm 67:3 Let the people (___) praise thee, O God; let all the people (___) praise thee.

WORSHIP
<u>**Promise 10**</u> **John 4:23-24** But the hour cometh, and now is, when the true worshippers (____) shall worship the Father in spirit and in truth: for the Father seeketh such (____) to worship him. God is a spirit: and they (____) that worship him must worship him in spirit and in truth.

Psalm 95:6 O come, let us (____) worship and bow down: let us (____) kneel before the Lord our maker.

Philippians 3:3 For we (____) are the circumcision, which worship God in the spirit, and rejoice in Christ Jesus, and have no confidence in the flesh.

Revelation 19:10 And I (____) fell at his feet to worship him.

Psalm 99:5 Exalt ye (____) the Lord our God, and worship at his footstool; for he is holy.

Matthew 4:10 Thou (____) shalt worship the Lord thy God, and him only shalt thou (____) serve.

EARLY & LATTER RAIN

<u>Promise 11</u>   **James 5:7-8**   Be patient therefore, brethren (___), unto the coming of the Lord. Behold, the husbandman (Our Father) waiteth for the precious fruit (souls) of the earth, and hath long patience for it, until he receive the early and latter rain. Be ye also patient (___); stablish your (___) hearts: for the coming of the Lord draweth nigh.

Acts 2:16-17   But this is (the beginning of) that which was spoken by the prophet Joel; And it shall come to pass in the last days, saith God, I will pour out of my Spirit upon all flesh (___): and your (___) sons and your (___) daughters shall prophesy, and your young men (___) shall see visions, and your old men (___) shall dream dreams.

Zechariah 10:1   Ask ye (___) of the Lord rain in the time of the latter rain.

Hosea 6:3   He (Holy Spirit) shall come unto us (___) as the rain, as the latter and former rain unto the earth.

GLORY - GOD'S PRESENCE - WORSHIP
<u>Promise 12</u>   **John 17:22**   And the glory which
thou gavest me I (Jesus) have given them (___);
that they (___) may be one, even as we are one.

II Corinthians 3:18   But we all (___), with open
face beholding as in a glass the glory of the Lord,
are changed into the same image from glory to
glory, even as by the Spirit of the Lord.

Leviticus 9:6   And Moses said, This is the thing
(worship) which the Lord commanded ye (___)
should do: and the glory of the Lord shall appear
unto you (___).

Isaiah 6:3   Holy, holy, holy, is the Lord of hosts:
the whole earth is full of his glory.

Psalm 29:2-3   Give (___) unto the Lord the glory
due unto his name; (___) worship the Lord in the
beauty of holiness. The voice of the Lord is upon
the waters: the God of glory thundereth: the Lord
is upon many waters.

FAITH
<u>Promise 13</u>   **Romans 10:17**   So then faith
(____faith) cometh by hearing, and hearing by the
word of God.

Matthew 21:22   And all things, whatsoever ye
(___) shall ask in prayer, believing, ye (___) shall
receive.

II Corinthians 5:7   For we (___) walk by faith,
not by sight.

Hebrews 11:1 & 3 & 6   Now faith is the
substance of things hoped for, the evidence of
things not seen.   Through faith we (___)
understand that the worlds were framed by the
word of God, so that things which are seen were
not made of things which do appear. But without
faith it is impossible to please him: for he (___)
that cometh to God must believe that he is, and that
he is a rewarder of them (___) that diligently seek
him.

Mark 11:24 Therefore I say unto you (___), What
things soever ye (___) desire, when ye (___) pray,
believe that ye (___) receive them, and ye (___)
shall have them.

HEALING

Promise 14 **I Peter 2:24** Who his own self bare our (___) sins in his own body on the tree, that we (___), being dead to sins, should live unto righteousness: by whose stripes ye (___) were healed.

Psalm 107:20 He sent his word (Jesus, Bible), and healed them (___), and delivered them (___) from their destructions.

Matthew 8:16-17 When the even was come, they brought unto him (Jesus) many that were possessed with devils: and he (Jesus) cast out the spirits with his word, and healed all that were sick: That it might be fulfilled which was spoken by Isaiah the prophet, saying, Himself (Jesus) took our (___) infirmities, and bare our (___) sicknesses.

Exodus 23:25 And ye (___) shall serve the Lord your (___) God, and he shall bless thy (___) bread, and thy (___) water; and I will take sickness away from the midst of thee (___).

HEALING

Promise 15 Isaiah 53:4-5 Surely he (Jesus) hath borne our (___) griefs, and carried our (___) sorrows: yet we (___) did esteem him (Jesus) stricken, smitten of God, and afflicted. But he (Jesus) was wounded for our (___) transgressions, he (Jesus) was bruised for our (___) iniquities: the chastisement of our (___) peace was upon him (Jesus); and with his (Jesus') stripes we (___) are healed.

Job 33:25 His (___) flesh shall be fresher than a child's: he (___) shall return to the days of his youth.

Psalm 30:2 O Lord my (___) God, I (___) cried unto thee, and thou hast healed me (___).

Psalm 103:3 Who forgiveth all thine (___) iniquities; who healeth all thy (___) diseases.

John 10:10 The thief (Satan, demons) cometh not, but for to steal, and to kill, and to destroy: I (Jesus) am come that they (___) might have life, and that they (___) might have it more abundantly.

PROTECTION
<u>Promise 16</u>   **Psalm 91:1-16**   He (___) that
dwelleth in the secret place of the most High shall
abide under the shadow of the Almighty. I (___)
will say of the Lord, He is my (___) refuge and my
(___) fortress: my (___) God; in him will I (___)
trust. Surely he shall deliver thee (___) from the
snare of the fowler, and from the noisome
pestilence. He shall cover thee (___) with his
feathers, and under his wings shalt thou (___)
trust: his truth shall be thy (___) shield and
buckler. Thou (___) shalt not be afraid for the
terror by night; nor for the arrow that flieth by day;
Nor for the pestilence that walketh in darkness; nor
for the destruction that wasteth at noonday. A
thousand shall fall at thy (___) side, and ten
thousand at thy (___) right hand; but it shall not
come nigh thee (___). Only with thine (___) eyes
shalt thou (___) behold and see the reward of the
wicked. Because thou (___) hast made the Lord,
which is my (___) refuge, even the most High, thy
(___) habitation; There shall no evil befall thee
(___), neither shall any plague come nigh thy (___)
dwelling. For he shall give his angels charge over
thee (___), to keep thee (___) in all thy ways.

PROTECTION

They shall bear thee (___) up in their hands, lest thou dash thy (___) foot against a stone. Thou (___) shalt tread upon the lion and adder: the young lion and the dragon shalt thou (___) trample under feet. Because He (___) hath set his love upon me, therefore will I deliver him (___): I will set him (___) on high, because he hath known my name. He (___) shall call upon me, and I will answer him (___): I will be with him (___) in trouble; I will deliver him (___), and honour him (___). With long life will I satisfy him (___), and show him (___) my salvation.

Hebrews 4:14-16 Seeing then that we (___) have a great high priest, that is passed into the heavens, Jesus the Son of God, let us (___) hold fast our (___) profession (confession). For we (___) have not an high priest which cannot be touched with the feeling of our (___) infirmities; but was in all points tempted like as we (___) are, yet without sin. Let us (___) therefore come boldly unto the throne of grace (God), that we (___) may obtain mercy, and find grace (God's ability) to help in time of need.

DELIVERANCE

Promise 17   **Luke 10:19** Behold, I give unto you (___) power to tread on serpents and scorpions, and over all the power of the enemy: and nothing shall by any means hurt you (___).

Mark 16:17-18 ...In my name (Jesus) shall they (___) cast out devils; they (___) shall speak with new tongues;... they (___) shall lay hands on the sick, and they shall recover.

Philippians 2:9-11   Wherefore God also hath highly exalted him (Jesus), and given him (Jesus) a name which is above every name (all names): That at the name of Jesus every knee should bow (sickness, bondage, etc.), of things in heaven, things in earth, and things under the earth; And that every tongue (___) should confess that Jesus Christ is Lord, to the glory of God the Father.

Colossians 2:10   And ye (___) are complete in him (Jesus), which is the head of all principality and power:

GOD NEVER CHANGES
Promise 18   **Jeremiah 33:3**   Call unto me (Father, Jesus, Holy Spirit) and I will answer thee (___), and show thee (___) great and mighty things, which thou (___) knowest not.

II Corinthians 5:17-19   Therefore if any man (___) be in Christ, he (___) is a new creature: old things are passed away; behold, all things are become new. And all things are of God, who hath reconciled us (___) to himself by Jesus Christ, and hath given to us (___) the ministry of reconciliation; To wit, that God was in Christ, reconciling the world unto himself, not imputing their trespasses unto them (___); and hath committed unto us (___) the word of reconciliation.

Romans 2:11   For there is no respect of persons (___) with God.

Malachi 3:6   For I am the Lord, I change not.

Hebrews 13:8   Jesus Christ the same yesterday, and to day, and for ever.

BLESSINGS

<u>Promise 19</u> **Deuteronomy 28:1-14** And it shall come to pass, if thou (___) shalt hearken diligently unto the voice of the Lord thy God, to observe and to do all his commandments (Word) which I command thee (___) this day, that the Lord thy God will set thee (___) on high above all nations of the earth: And all these blessings shall come on thee (___), and overtake thee (___), if thou (___) shalt hearken unto the voice of the Lord thy God. Blessed shalt thou (___) be in the city, and blessed shalt thou (___) be in the field. Blessed shalt be the fruit of thy (___) body (children), and the fruit of thy (___) ground, and the fruit of thy (___) cattle, the increase of thy (___) kine, and the flocks of thy (·___) sheep. Blessed shall be thy (___) basket and thy (___) store. Blessed shalt thou (___) be when thou (___) comest in, and blessed shalt thou (___) be when thou (___) goest out. The Lord shall cause thine (___) enemies that rise up against thee (___) to be smitten before thy (___) face: they shall come out against thee (___) one way, and flee before thee (___) seven ways. The Lord shall command the blessing upon thee (___) in thy (___) storehouses, and in all thou

30

BLESSINGS

(___) settest thine (___) hand unto; and he shall
bless thee(___) in the land which the Lord thy God
giveth thee (___). The Lord shall establish thee
(___) an holy people unto himself, as he hath
sworn unto thee (___), if thou (___) shalt keep the
commandments of the Lord thy God, and walk in
his ways. And all people of the earth shall see that
thou (___) art called by the name of the Lord
(Jesus); and they shall be afraid of thee (___). And
the Lord shall make thee (___) plenteous in goods,
in the fruit of thy (___) body, and in the fruit of thy
(___) cattle, and in the fruit of thy (___) ground, in
the land which the Lord sware unto thy fathers to
give thee. The Lord shall open unto thee (___) his
good treasure, the heaven to give the rain unto thy
(___) land in his season, and to bless all the work
of thine (___) hand: and thou shalt lend unto many
nations, and thou (___) shalt not borrow. And the
Lord shall make thee (___) the head, and not the
tail; and thou (___) shalt be above only, and thou
(___) shalt not be beneath; if that thou (___)
hearken unto the commandments of the Lord thy
God, which I command thee (___) this day, to

BLESSINGS

observe and to do them: And thou (___) shalt not go aside from any of the words which I command thee (___) this day, to the right hand, or to the left, to go after other gods to serve them.

Galatians 3:13-15 Christ hath redeemed us (___) from the curse of the law, being made a curse for us (___): for it is written, Cursed is every one that hangeth on a tree: That the blessing of Abraham might come on the Gentiles (___) through Jesus Christ; that we (___) might receive the promise of the Spirit through faith.

II Corinthians 1:20 For all the promises of God in him (Jesus) are yea (yes), and in him (Jesus) Amen (so be it), unto the glory of God by us.

II Timothy 3:16-17 All scripture is given by inspiration of God, and is profitable for (___) doctrine, for reproof, for correction, for instruction in righteousness: That the man of God (___) may be perfect, thoroughly furnished unto all good works.

HOLY SPIRIT
<u>Promise 20</u> **John 14:16-17** And I (Jesus) will pray the Father, and he shall give you (___) another Comforter, that he may abide with you (___) **for ever**; Even the Spirit of truth; whom the world (unsaved) cannot receive, because it seeth him not, neither knoweth him: but ye (___) know him; for he dwelleth **with you** (___), and shall be **in you** (___).

Luke 11:11-13 If a son shall ask bread of any of you that is a father, will he give him a stone? or if he ask a fish, will he for a fish give him a serpent? Or if he shall ask an egg, will he offer him a scorpion? If ye then, being evil, know how to give good gifts unto your children: how much more shall your heavenly Father give the Holy Spirit to them (___) that ask him?

Acts 1:8 But ye (___) shall receive power, after that the Holy Ghost is come upon you (___).

Acts 24 And they were all filled with the Holy Ghost, and (they) (___) began to speak with other tongues, as the Spirit gave them utterance.

HOLY SPIRIT
<u>Promise 21</u>   **John 14:26**   But the Comforter, which is the Holy Ghost (Holy Spirit), whom the Father will send in my name, he shall teach you (___) all things, and bring all things to your (___) remembrance, whatsoever I have said unto you.

John 15:26   But when the Comforter is come, whom I will send unto you (___) from the Father, even the Spirit of truth, which proceedeth from the Father, he shall testify of me (Jesus).

John 16:13   Howbeit when he, the Spirit of truth, is come, he will guide you (___) into all truth: for he shall not speak of himself; but whatsoever he shall hear, that shall he speak: and he (Holy Spirit) will show you (___) **things to come**.

Romans 8:26-27   Likewise the Spirit also helpeth our (___) infirmities: for we (___) know not what we (___) should pray for as we (___) ought: but the Spirit itself maketh intercession for us (___) with groanings which cannot be uttered. And he that searcheth the hearts knoweth what is the mind of the Spirit, because he maketh intercession for the saints (___) according to the will of God.

HOLY SPIRIT

Promise 22 **Romans 8:11** But if the Spirit of him that raised up Jesus from the dead dwell in you (___), he that raised up Christ from the dead shall also quicken your (___) mortal (death doomed) bodies by his Spirit that dwelleth in you (___).

I Corinthians 14:4 He (___) that speaketh in an unknown tongue edifieth himself (___).

Jude 20 But ye (___), beloved, building up yourselves (___) on your (___) most holy faith, praying in the Holy Ghost.

I Corinthians 12:8-10 For to one (___) is given by the Spirit the word of wisdom; to another (___) the word of knowledge by the same Spirit; To another (___) faith by the same Spirit; to another (___) the gifts of healing by the same Spirit; to another (___) the working of miracles; to another (___) prophecy; to another (___) discerning of spirits; to another (___) divers kinds of tongues; to another (___) the interpretation of tongues.

PEACE

<u>Promise 23</u>   **John 14:27**   Peace I (Jesus) leave with you (___), my peace I give unto you (___): not as the world giveth, give I unto you (___). Let not your (___) heart be troubled, neither let it be afraid.

John 16:33   In me (Jesus) ye (___) might have peace. In the world ye (___) shall have tribulation: but be of good cheer; I (Jesus) have overcome the world.

Matthew 11:28-30   Come unto me (Jesus), all ye (___) that labor and are heavy laden, and I (Jesus) will give you (___) rest. Take my yoke upon you (___), and learn of me; for I am meek and lowly in heart: and ye (___) shall find rest unto your (___) souls. For my yoke is easy, and my burden is light.

Isaiah 26:3   Thou wilt keep him (___) in perfect peace, whose mind is stayed on thee (Jesus): because he (___) trusteth in thee (Jesus).

WORRY-ANXIETY

<u>Promise 24</u> **Philippians 4:6** (___) Be careful (anxious, worried, fretting, upset) for nothing.

II Corinthians 10:5 (___) Casting down imaginations (thoughts, reasoning, wondering), and every high thing that exalteth itself against the knowledge (Word) of God, and bringing into captivity every thought to the obedience of Christ.

I Peter 5:6-9 Humble yourselves (___) therefore under the mighty hand of God, that he may exalt you (___) in due time: Casting all your (___) cares (worries, anxieties) upon him; for he careth for you (___). Be sober, be vigilant; because your (___) adversary the devil, as a roaring lion, walketh about, seeking whom he may devour: Whom (___) resist stedfast in the faith.

Matthew 6:33-34 But seek ye (___) first the kingdom of God, and his righteousness; and all these things shall be added unto you (___). Take therefore no thought (anxious thought) for the morrow: for the morrow shall take thought for the things of itself. Sufficient unto the day is the evil thereof.

LOVE

<u>Promise 25</u> **I Corinthians 13:4-8** Charity (God kind of love) suffereth long, and is kind; charity (love) envieth not; charity (love) vaunteth not itself, is not puffed up, Doth not behave itself unseemly, seeketh not her own, is not easily provoked, thinketh no evil; Rejoiceth not in iniquity, but rejoiceth in the truth; Beareth all things, believeth all things, hopeth all things, endureth all things. Charity (love) never faileth.

I John 4:18 There is no fear in love; but perfect love (God's love) casteth out fear: because fear hath torment. He (___) that feareth is not made perfect in love.

Luke 10:27 And he (Jesus) answering said, Thou (___) shalt love the Lord thy (___) God with all thy (___) heart, and with all thy (___) soul, and with all thy (___) strength, and with all thy (___) mind; and thy (___) neighbor as thyself.

Romans 5:5 The love of God is shed abroad in our (___) hearts by the Holy Ghost which is given unto us (___).

STRENGTH

<u>Promise 26</u> **Philippians 4:13** I (___) can do all things through Christ which strengtheneth me.

Joel 3:10 Let the weak (___) say, I (___) am strong.

Romans 4:20 He (___) staggered not at the promise of God through unbelief; but was **strong** in faith, giving glory (praise, worship) to God.

Psalm 27:1 The Lord is my (___) light and my (___) salvation; whom shall I (___) fear? the Lord is the **strength** of my (___) life; of whom shall I (___) be afraid?

Psalm 29:11 The Lord will give **strength** unto his people (___); the Lord will bless his people (___) with peace.

Psalm 46:1 God is our (___) refuge and strength, a very present help in trouble.

JOY

<u>Promise 27</u> **Nehemiah 8:10** The joy of the Lord is your (___) strength.

John 16:23-24 And in that day ye (___) shall ask me (Jesus) nothing, Verily, verily, I say unto you (___), Whatsoever ye (___) shall ask the Father in my (Jesus) name, he will give it you (___). Hitherto have ye (___) asked nothing in my name: ask, and ye (___) shall receive, that your (___) **joy** may be full.

Psalm 16:11 Thou wilt show me (___) the path of life: in thy presence is fulness of **joy**; at thy right hand there are pleasures for evermore.

Psalm 51:12 Restore unto me (___) the joy of thy salvation; and uphold me (___) with thy free spirit.

Ecclesiastes 2:26 For God giveth to a man (___) that is good in his sight wisdom, and knowledge, and **joy**.

COME BEFORE GOD'S THRONE

Promise 28 **Hebrews 4:16** Let us (___) therefore come boldly unto the throne of grace (God), that we (___) may obtain mercy, and find grace (God's ability) to help in time of need.

Psalm 91:1 He (___) that dwelleth in the secret place of the most High (before God's throne) shall abide under the shadow of the Almighty.

Matthew 6:11 Give us (___) this day our (___) daily bread.

Matthew 7:7 Ask, and it shall be given you (___); seek, and ye (___) shall find; knock, and it shall be opened unto you (___).

Psalm 46:10 Be still (___), and know that I am God.

Isaiah 40:31 But they (___) that wait upon the Lord shall renew their (___) strength; they (___) shall mount up with wings as eagles; they (___) shall run, and not be weary; and they (___) shall walk, and not faint.

PROSPERITY

<u>Promise 29</u> **III John 2** Beloved, I wish above all things that thou (____) mayest prosper and be in health, even as thy (____) soul prospereth.

Deuteronomy 8:18 But thou (____) shalt remember the Lord thy (____) God: for it is he that giveth thee (____) power to get wealth, that he may establish his covenant which he sware unto thy (____) fathers.

Luke 6:38 Give, and it shall be given unto you (____); good measure, pressed down, and shaken together, and running over, shall men give into your (____) bosom. For with the same measure that ye (____) mete withal it shall be measured to you (____) again.

Proverbs 10:22 The blessing of the Lord, it maketh (____) rich.

Mark 10:30 But he (____) shall receive a hundredfold now in this time, houses, and brethren, and sisters, and mothers, and children, and lands, with persecutions; and in the world to come eternal life.

WISDOM

<u>Promise 30</u> **James 1:5** If any of you (___) lack wisdom, let him (___) ask of God, that giveth to all men (___) liberally, and upbraideth not; and it shall be given him (___).

Proverbs 2:2 & 6 So that thou (___) incline thine ear unto wisdom, and apply thine heart to understanding. For the Lord giveth wisdom: out of his mouth cometh knowledge and understanding.

Proverbs 3:13 Happy is the man (___) that findeth wisdom, and the man (___) that getteth understanding.

Proverbs 16:16 How much better is it to get wisdom (___) than gold! and to get understanding rather to be chosen than silver!

I Corinthians 1:30 But of him are ye (___) in Christ Jesus, who of God is made unto us (___) wisdom, and righteousness, and sanctification, and redemption.

SEATED WITH CHRIST JESUS
<u>Promise 31</u>   **Psalm 27:14** Wait on the Lord: be
of good courage, and he shall strengthen thine
(___) heart: wait, I say, on the Lord.

Psalm 34:7 The angel of the Lord encampeth
round about them (___) that fear him, and
delivereth them (___).

Psalm 34:9-10 O fear (reverence) the Lord, ye
(___) his saints: for there is no want to them (___)
that fear him. They (___) that seek the Lord shall
not want any good thing.

Psalm 34:17 The righteous (___) cry, and the
Lord heareth, and delivereth them (___) out of all
their troubles.

Ephesians 2:6-7 And hath raised us (___) up
together, and made us (___) sit together in
heavenly places in Christ Jesus: That in the ages to
come he might show the exceeding riches of his
grace in his kindness toward us (___) through
Christ Jesus.

COMMITMENT

<u>Promise 32</u> **Psalm 37:3-7** Trust in the Lord, and do good; so shalt thou (___) dwell in the land, and verily thou (___) shalt be fed. Delight thyself (___) also in the Lord; and he shall give thee (___) the desires of thine (___) heart. Commit thy (___) way unto the Lord; trust also in him; and he shall bring it to pass. And he shall bring forth thy (___) righteousness as the light, and thy (___) judgment as the noonday. Rest in the Lord, and wait patiently for him: fret not thyself (___) because of him who prospereth in his way, because of the man who bringeth wicked devices to pass.

Psalm 37:23 The steps of a good man (___) are ordered by the Lord: and he delighteth in his (___) way.

Colossians 3:17 And whatsoever ye (___) do in word or deed, do all in the name of the Lord Jesus, giving thanks to God and the Father by him.

<u>**Promise 33**</u> **Ephesians 1:17-23** That the God of our (___) Lord Jesus Christ, the Father of glory, may give unto you (___) the spirit of wisdom and revelation in the knowledge of him: The eyes of your (___) understanding being enlightened; that ye (___) may know what is the hope of his calling, and what the riches of the glory of his inheritance in the saints. And what is the exceeding greatness of his power to usward (___) who believe, according to the working of his mighty power, Which he wrought in Christ, when he raised him from the dead, and set him at his own right hand in the heavenly places, Far above all principality, and power, and might, and dominion, and every name that is named, not only in this world, but also in that which is to come: And hath put all things under his feet, and gave him to be the head over all things to the church, Which is his body, the fullness of him that filleth all in all.

John 1:4 In him (Jesus) was life; and the life was the light of men (___).

I Peter 2:9 Him (Jesus) who hath called you (___) out of darkness into his marvellous light.

46

Promise 34 **Ephesians 3:14-21** For this cause I (___) bow my (___) knees unto the Father of our (___) Lord Jesus Christ, Of whom the whole family in heaven and earth is named, That he would grant you (___), according to the riches of his glory, to be strengthened with might by his Spirit in the (my) inner man; That Christ may dwell in your (___) hearts by faith; that ye (___) being rooted and grounded in love, May be able to comprehend with all saints what is the breadth, and length, and depth, and height; And to know the love of Christ, which passeth knowledge, that ye (___) might be filled with all the fullness of God. Now unto him that is able to do exceeding abundantly above all that we ask or think, according to the power that worketh in us (___), Unto him be glory in the church by Christ Jesus throughout all ages, world without end.

Psalm 112:1-3 Praise ye (___) the Lord. Blessed is the man (___) that feareth the Lord, that delighteth greatly in his commandments. His seed (children) shall be mighty upon earth: the generation of the upright shall be blessed. Wealth and riches shall be in his (___) house: and his righteousness endureth for ever.

PLEASING GOD
<u>Promise 35</u>   **Proverbs 3:9-10** Honor the Lord
with thy (___) substance, and with the first fruits
of all thine (___) increase: So shall thy (___) barns
be filled with plenty, and thy (___) presses shall
burst out with new wine.

James 4:7 Submit yourselves (___) therefore to
God. Resist the devil, and he will flee from you
(___).

Proverbs 10:11 The mouth of a righteous man
(___) is a well of life: but violence covereth the
mouth of the wicked (unrighteous).

Proverbs 16:7 When a man's (___) ways please
the Lord, he maketh even his (___) enemies to be
at peace with him.

John 6:63   (Jesus said) It is the spirit that
quickeneth; the flesh profiteth nothing: the words
that I speak unto you (___), they are spirit, and
they are life.

48

DOING GOD'S WORD
<u>Promise 36</u> **James 1:22** But be ye (___) doers of the word (Bible), and not hearers only, deceiving your own selves (___).

Proverbs 21:23 Whoso (___) keepeth his (___) mouth and his (___) tongue keepeth his soul from troubles.

Proverbs 29:25 The fear of man bringeth a snare: but whoso (___) putteth his (___) trust in the Lord shall be safe.

Isaiah 1:19 If ye (___) be willing and obedient, ye (___) shall eat the good of the land.

John 15:7 If ye (___) abide in me (Jesus), and my words abide in you (___), ye (___) shall ask what ye (___) will, and it shall be done unto you (___).

Psalm 119:89 For ever, O Lord, thy word is settled in heaven (and in my heart).